RATING

☆☆☆☆☆

· ·

PREP TIME

COOKING TIME

DIFFICULTY

OVEN TEMPERATURE

SOURCE

NUMBER OF SERVINGS

1 2 3 4 5 ....

°C

INGREDIENTS

_____

_____

_____

_____

_____

_____

_____

_____

METHOD

_____

_____

_____

_____

_____

_____

_____

_____

_____

_____

_____

_____

NOTES

_____

_____

_____

_____

_____

_____

_____

_____

_____

RECIPE ORIGIN

_____

RATING

☆☆☆☆☆

. . . .

:

PREP TIME

COOKING TIME

DIFFICULTY

○○○○○

OVEN TEMPERATURE

_____

SOURCE

_____

NUMBER OF SERVINGS

1 2 3 4 5 ....

°C

INGREDIENTS

METHOD

_____
_____
_____
_____
_____
_____

NOTES

_____
_____
_____

_____
_____
_____
_____
_____
_____

RECIPE ORIGIN

_____

RATING
☆☆☆☆☆

. . . .

PREP TIME

COOKING TIME

DIFFICULTY

OVEN TEMPERATURE

SOURCE

NUMBER OF SERVINGS

1 2 3 4 5 ....

°C

INGREDIENTS

METHOD

NOTES

RECIPE ORIGIN

RATING

☆☆☆☆☆

. . . .

PREP TIME

COOKING TIME

DIFFICULTY

OVEN TEMPERATURE

SOURCE

NUMBER OF SERVINGS

1 2 3 4 5 ....

°C

INGREDIENTS

_____

_____

_____

_____

_____

_____

_____

METHOD

_____

_____

_____

_____

_____

_____

_____

_____

_____

_____

NOTES

_____

_____

_____

_____

_____

_____

_____

_____

_____

_____

_____

RECIPE ORIGIN

_____

_____

RATING
☆☆☆☆☆

· ·

PREP TIME

:

COOKING TIME

DIFFICULTY
○○○○○

OVEN TEMPERATURE
____

SOURCE
____

NUMBER OF SERVINGS

1 2 3 4 5 ....

℃

INGREDIENTS
_____
_____
_____
_____
_____
_____
_____

METHOD
_____
_____
_____
_____
_____
_____
_____
_____
_____
_____
_____
_____
_____
_____

NOTES
_____
_____
_____
_____
_____
_____
_____
_____

__ __

RECIPE ORIGIN
_____

RATING

☆☆☆☆☆

∙∙

PREP TIME

COOKING TIME

DIFFICULTY

OVEN TEMPERATURE

SOURCE

NUMBER OF SERVINGS

1 2 3 4 5 ....

℃

INGREDIENTS

METHOD

NOTES

RECIPE ORIGIN

RATING

☆☆☆☆☆

· ·

PREP TIME

COOKING TIME

DIFFICULTY
○○○○○

OVEN TEMPERATURE

SOURCE

NUMBER OF SERVINGS

1 2 3 4 5 ....

°C

INGREDIENTS

_____

_____

_____

_____

_____

_____

_____

METHOD

_____

_____

_____

_____

_____

_____

_____

_____

_____

_____

_____

_____

_____

NOTES

_____

_____

_____

_____

_____

_____

RECIPE ORIGIN

_____

RATING

☆☆☆☆☆

. . . .

PREP TIME

COOKING TIME

DIFFICULTY

○○○○

OVEN TEMPERATURE

SOURCE

NUMBER OF SERVINGS

1 2 3 4 5 ....

℃

INGREDIENTS

METHOD

NOTES

RECIPE ORIGIN

RATING

☆☆☆☆☆

· ·

PREP TIME

COOKING TIME

DIFFICULTY
◉◉◉◉◉

OVEN TEMPERATURE

SOURCE
_____

°C

NUMBER OF SERVINGS

1 2 3 4 5 ....

INGREDIENTS

_____
_____
_____
_____
_____
_____
_____

METHOD

_____
_____
_____
_____
_____
_____
_____
_____
_____
_____
_____
_____
_____

NOTES

_____
_____
_____
_____
_____
_____

_____

RECIPE ORIGIN

_____

RATING

☆☆☆☆☆

....

PREP TIME

COOKING TIME

DIFFICULTY

OVEN TEMPERATURE

SOURCE

NUMBER OF SERVINGS

1 2 3 4 5 ....

°c

INGREDIENTS

METHOD

NOTES

RECIPE ORIGIN

RATING

☆☆☆☆☆

- -

PREP TIME

COOKING TIME

DIFFICULTY
○○○○○

OVEN TEMPERATURE

SOURCE
_____

NUMBER OF SERVINGS

1 2 3 4 5 ....

°C

INGREDIENTS

_____
_____
_____
_____
_____
_____
_____

_ _

RECIPE ORIGIN

_____

NOTES

_____
_____
_____
_____
_____

METHOD

_____
_____
_____
_____
_____
_____
_____
_____
_____
_____
_____
_____

RATING

☆☆☆☆☆

· ·

PREP TIME

COOKING TIME

DIFFICULTY
○○○○○

OVEN TEMPERATURE
_____

SOURCE
_____

NUMBER OF SERVINGS

1 2 3 4 5 ....

°C

METHOD

INGREDIENTS

_____
_____
_____
_____
_____
_____
_____

NOTES

RECIPE ORIGIN

_____

RATING

☆☆☆☆☆

....

PREP TIME

COOKING TIME

DIFFICULTY

OVEN TEMPERATURE

SOURCE

NUMBER OF SERVINGS

1 2 3 4 5 ....

°C

METHOD

INGREDIENTS

NOTES

RECIPE ORIGIN

RATING

☆☆☆☆☆

· ·

PREP TIME

:

COOKING TIME

DIFFICULTY

OVEN TEMPERATURE

SOURCE

NUMBER OF SERVINGS

1 2 3 4 5 ....

℃

INGREDIENTS

METHOD

NOTES

RECIPE ORIGIN

RATING

☆☆☆☆☆

⏰

PREP TIME

🕐

COOKING TIME

DIFFICULTY
● ● ● ● ●

OVEN TEMPERATURE

_____

SOURCE

_____

NUMBER OF SERVINGS

1 2 3 4 5 ....

°C

INGREDIENTS

_____

_____

_____

_____

_____

_____

_____

METHOD

_____

_____

_____

_____

_____

_____

_____

_____

_____

_____

_____

_____

📝

NOTES

_____

_____

_____

_____

_____

_____

RECIPE ORIGIN

_____

RATING
☆☆☆☆☆

· ·

:
PREP TIME

COOKING TIME

DIFFICULTY
◦ ◦ ◦ ◦

OVEN TEMPERATURE
_____

SOURCE
_____

NUMBER OF SERVINGS

1 2 3 4 5 ....

°C

INGREDIENTS
_____
_____
_____
_____
_____
_____
_____

_ _ _

RECIPE ORIGIN
_____

METHOD
_____
_____
_____
_____
_____
_____
_____
_____
_____
_____
_____
_____
_____
_____
_____

NOTES
_____
_____
_____
_____
_____
_____

RATING

☆☆☆☆☆

• •

PREP TIME

:

COOKING TIME

DIFFICULTY

⚫⚫⚫⚫⚫

OVEN TEMPERATURE

SOURCE

°C

NUMBER OF SERVINGS

1 2 3 4 5 ....

INGREDIENTS

METHOD

NOTES

RECIPE ORIGIN

RATING

☆☆☆☆☆

....

PREP TIME

COOKING TIME

DIFFICULTY
○○○○○

OVEN TEMPERATURE

SOURCE
‒‒‒‒‒‒

NUMBER OF SERVINGS

1 2 3 4 5 ....

℃

INGREDIENTS

_____

_____

_____

_____

_____

_____

METHOD

_____

_____

_____

_____

_____

_____

_____

_____

NOTES

_____

_____

_____

_____

_____

_____

‒ ‒

RECIPE ORIGIN
_____

RATING
☆☆☆☆☆

....

⏰
PREP TIME
:

🕐
COOKING TIME

👨‍🍳
DIFFICULTY
○○○○○

🍳
OVEN TEMPERATURE
___

SOURCE
___

NUMBER OF SERVINGS

1 2 3 4 5 ....

°C

INGREDIENTS

_____
_____
_____
_____
_____
_____
_____

METHOD

_____
_____
_____
_____
_____
_____
_____
_____
_____
_____

📝
NOTES

_____
_____
_____
_____
_____

RECIPE ORIGIN
_____

RATING
☆☆☆☆☆

....

PREP TIME

COOKING TIME

DIFFICULTY
○○○○○

OVEN TEMPERATURE
_____

SOURCE
_____

NUMBER OF SERVINGS

1 2 3 4 5 ....

°C

INGREDIENTS
_____
_____
_____
_____
_____
_____
_____

METHOD
_____
_____
_____
_____
_____
_____
_____
_____
_____
_____
_____
_____

NOTES
_____
_____
_____
_____
_____
_____

— —

RECIPE ORIGIN
_____

RATING

☆☆☆☆☆

....

PREP TIME

COOKING TIME

DIFFICULTY
●●●●●

OVEN TEMPERATURE

SOURCE

NUMBER OF SERVINGS

1 2 3 4 5 ....

°C

INGREDIENTS

METHOD

NOTES

RECIPE ORIGIN

RATING
☆☆☆☆☆

. . . .

PREP TIME

COOKING TIME

DIFFICULTY
○○○○○

OVEN TEMPERATURE
_____

SOURCE
_____

NUMBER OF SERVINGS

1 2 3 4 5 ....

℃

INGREDIENTS
_____
_____
_____
_____
_____
_____
_____
_____

METHOD
_____
_____
_____
_____
_____
_____
_____
_____
_____
_____
_____
_____

NOTES
_____
_____
_____
_____
_____
_____
_____
_____
_____

___ ___

RECIPE ORIGIN
_____

RATING

☆☆☆☆☆

- -

PREP TIME

COOKING TIME

DIFFICULTY
⬤⬤⬤⬤⬤

OVEN TEMPERATURE

SOURCE

°C

NUMBER OF SERVINGS

1 2 3 4 5 ....

INGREDIENTS

METHOD

NOTES

RECIPE ORIGIN

RATING
☆☆☆☆☆

. . . .

PREP TIME

COOKING TIME

DIFFICULTY
○○○○○

OVEN TEMPERATURE
_____

SOURCE
_____

NUMBER OF SERVINGS

1 2 3 4 5 ....

℃

INGREDIENTS
_____
_____
_____
_____
_____
_____
_____

METHOD
_____
_____
_____
_____
_____
_____
_____
_____

NOTES
_____
_____
_____
_____
_____
_____
_____
_____

__ __

RECIPE ORIGIN
_____

RATING

☆☆☆☆☆

· ·

PREP TIME

COOKING TIME

DIFFICULTY

OVEN TEMPERATURE

SOURCE

_____

NUMBER OF SERVINGS

1 2 3 4 5 ....

°C

INGREDIENTS

_____

_____

_____

_____

_____

_____

_____

_ _

RECIPE ORIGIN

_____

METHOD

_____

_____

_____

_____

_____

_____

_____

_____

_____

_____

_____

_____

NOTES

_____

_____

_____

_____

_____

RATING

☆☆☆☆☆

· ·

PREP TIME

:

COOKING TIME

DIFFICULTY

OVEN TEMPERATURE

SOURCE

NUMBER OF SERVINGS

1 2 3 4 5 ....

°C

METHOD

INGREDIENTS

NOTES

RECIPE ORIGIN

RATING

☆☆☆☆☆

- -

PREP TIME

COOKING TIME

DIFFICULTY

OVEN TEMPERATURE

SOURCE

NUMBER OF SERVINGS

1 2 3 4 5 ....

°c

INGREDIENTS

METHOD

NOTES

RECIPE ORIGIN

RATING

☆☆☆☆☆

· ·

PREP TIME

COOKING TIME

DIFFICULTY

OVEN TEMPERATURE

SOURCE

NUMBER OF SERVINGS

1 2 3 4 5 ....

°C

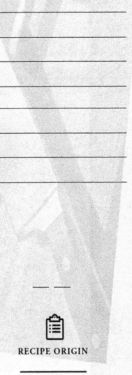

INGREDIENTS

RECIPE ORIGIN

NOTES

METHOD

RATING

☆☆☆☆☆

PREP TIME

COOKING TIME

DIFFICULTY
○○○○○

OVEN TEMPERATURE

SOURCE

NUMBER OF SERVINGS

1 2 3 4 5 ....

℃

INGREDIENTS

METHOD

NOTES

RECIPE ORIGIN

RATING
☆☆☆☆☆

· ·

PREP TIME

COOKING TIME

DIFFICULTY

OVEN TEMPERATURE

SOURCE

NUMBER OF SERVINGS

1 2 3 4 5 ....

°C

INGREDIENTS

METHOD

NOTES

RECIPE ORIGIN

RATING
☆☆☆☆☆

....

PREP TIME

COOKING TIME

DIFFICULTY
○○○○○

OVEN TEMPERATURE

SOURCE
_____

NUMBER OF SERVINGS

1 2 3 4 5 ....

°C

INGREDIENTS
_____
_____
_____
_____
_____
_____
_____
_____

METHOD
_____
_____
_____
_____
_____
_____
_____
_____
_____
_____
_____
_____
_____

NOTES
_____
_____
_____
_____
_____
_____

RECIPE ORIGIN
_____

RATING

☆☆☆☆☆

· ·

PREP TIME

COOKING TIME

DIFFICULTY

○○○○○

OVEN TEMPERATURE

SOURCE

NUMBER OF SERVINGS

1 2 3 4 5 ....

℃

INGREDIENTS

METHOD

_____

_____

_____

_____

_____

_____

NOTES

_____

_____

_____

_____

_____

_____

RECIPE ORIGIN

RATING
☆☆☆☆☆

· ·

PREP TIME

COOKING TIME

DIFFICULTY
○○○○

OVEN TEMPERATURE
_____

SOURCE
_____

NUMBER OF SERVINGS

1 2 3 4 5 ....

°C

METHOD

_____
_____
_____

INGREDIENTS

_____
_____
_____
_____
_____
_____
_____

_____
_____
_____
_____

NOTES

_____
_____
_____

_____
_____

— —

_____
_____

RECIPE ORIGIN

_____

_____
_____
_____
_____
_____

RATING

☆☆☆☆☆

• •

DIFFICULTY

○○○○○

PREP TIME

COOKING TIME

OVEN TEMPERATURE

SOURCE

°C

NUMBER OF SERVINGS

1 2 3 4 5 ....

METHOD

INGREDIENTS

_____

_____

_____

_____

_____

_____

_____

_____

NOTES

_____

_____

_____

_____

_____

_____

_____

_____

RECIPE ORIGIN

RATING

☆☆☆☆☆

....

PREP TIME

COOKING TIME

DIFFICULTY
○○○○○

OVEN TEMPERATURE
_____

SOURCE
_____

NUMBER OF SERVINGS

1 2 3 4 5 ....

°C

INGREDIENTS
_____
_____
_____
_____
_____
_____
_____

___ ___

RECIPE ORIGIN
_____

METHOD
_____
_____
_____
_____
_____
_____
_____
_____
_____
_____
_____
_____
_____
_____
_____

NOTES
_____
_____
_____
_____
_____
_____
_____
_____

RATING
☆☆☆☆☆

....

PREP TIME

COOKING TIME

DIFFICULTY
○○○○○

OVEN TEMPERATURE
_____

SOURCE
_____

NUMBER OF SERVINGS

1 2 3 4 5 ....

°C

INGREDIENTS
_____
_____
_____
_____
_____
_____
_____

METHOD
_____
_____
_____
_____
_____
_____
_____
_____
_____
_____
_____
_____
_____

NOTES
_____
_____
_____
_____
_____
_____
_____
_____

_ _ _

RECIPE ORIGIN
_____

RATING
☆☆☆☆☆

· ·

PREP TIME

COOKING TIME

DIFFICULTY
○○○○○

OVEN TEMPERATURE

SOURCE

NUMBER OF SERVINGS

1 2 3 4 5 ....

°C

INGREDIENTS

METHOD

NOTES

RECIPE ORIGIN

RATING

☆☆☆☆☆

....

PREP TIME

:

COOKING TIME

DIFFICULTY

○○○○○

OVEN TEMPERATURE

_____

°C

SOURCE

_____

NUMBER OF SERVINGS

1 2 3 4 5 ....

INGREDIENTS

_____
_____
_____
_____
_____
_____
_____

METHOD

_____
_____
_____
_____
_____
_____
_____
_____
_____
_____
_____
_____
_____
_____
_____
_____

NOTES

_____
_____
_____
_____
_____
_____

— —

RECIPE ORIGIN

_____

RATING
☆☆☆☆☆

⏰
:
PREP TIME

🕐
COOKING TIME

DIFFICULTY
⬤⬤⬤⬤

OVEN TEMPERATURE
____

SOURCE
____

NUMBER OF SERVINGS

1 2 3 4 5 ....

METHOD

INGREDIENTS
_____
_____
_____
_____
_____
_____
_____

NOTES
_____
_____
_____
_____
_____
_____

__ __
RECIPE ORIGIN
_____

°C

RATING
☆☆☆☆☆

· ·

PREP TIME

COOKING TIME

DIFFICULTY
● ● ● ● ●

OVEN TEMPERATURE

SOURCE

NUMBER OF SERVINGS

1 2 3 4 5 ....

°C

INGREDIENTS

METHOD

NOTES

RECIPE ORIGIN

RATING

☆☆☆☆☆

....

PREP TIME

COOKING TIME

DIFFICULTY
○○○○○

OVEN TEMPERATURE

°C

SOURCE

NUMBER OF SERVINGS

1 2 3 4 5 ....

INGREDIENTS

METHOD

NOTES

RECIPE ORIGIN

RATING

☆☆☆☆☆

....

🕰️
:
PREP TIME

🕐
COOKING TIME

👨‍🍳
DIFFICULTY
⚪⚪⚪⚪

🍃
SOURCE
_____

🍳
OVEN TEMPERATURE
_____

NUMBER OF SERVINGS

1 2 3 4 5 ....

°C

INGREDIENTS

_____
_____
_____
_____
_____
_____
_____
_____

— —

📋
RECIPE ORIGIN

_____

📝
NOTES

_____
_____
_____
_____
_____
_____
_____
_____

METHOD

_____
_____
_____
_____
_____
_____
_____
_____
_____
_____
_____
_____
_____
_____

RATING
☆☆☆☆☆

. . . .

PREP TIME

COOKING TIME

DIFFICULTY
●●●●●

OVEN TEMPERATURE
_____

SOURCE
_____

NUMBER OF SERVINGS

1 2 3 4 5 ....

°C

INGREDIENTS

_____
_____
_____
_____
_____
_____
_____

METHOD

_____
_____
_____
_____
_____
_____
_____
_____
_____
_____
_____

NOTES

_____
_____
_____
_____
_____
_____
_____

__ __

RECIPE ORIGIN

_____

RATING

☆☆☆☆☆

....

PREP TIME

COOKING TIME

DIFFICULTY

OVEN TEMPERATURE

SOURCE
_____

NUMBER OF SERVINGS

1 2 3 4 5 ....

°C

INGREDIENTS

_____

_____

_____

_____

_____

_____

_____

METHOD

_____

_____

_____

_____

_____

_____

_____

NOTES

_____

_____

_____

_____

_____

_____

___ ___

RECIPE ORIGIN

_____

_____

_____

_____

RATING

☆☆☆☆☆

....

PREP TIME

COOKING TIME

DIFFICULTY
○○○○○

OVEN TEMPERATURE

SOURCE

NUMBER OF SERVINGS

1 2 3 4 5 ....

°C

INGREDIENTS

_____
_____
_____
_____
_____
_____
_____

METHOD

_____
_____
_____
_____
_____
_____
_____
_____
_____
_____
_____

NOTES

_____
_____
_____
_____
_____
_____
_____
_____

RECIPE ORIGIN

_____

RATING

☆☆☆☆☆

....

🕰️

PREP TIME

:

🕐

COOKING TIME

DIFFICULTY

○○○○○

🍳

OVEN TEMPERATURE

_____

SOURCE

_____

NUMBER OF SERVINGS

1 2 3 4 5 ....

°C

INGREDIENTS

_____
_____
_____
_____
_____
_____
_____

— —

📋

RECIPE ORIGIN

_____

METHOD

_____
_____
_____
_____
_____
_____
_____
_____
_____
_____
_____
_____

📝

NOTES

_____
_____
_____
_____
_____
_____
_____

RATING
☆☆☆☆☆

- -

PREP TIME

COOKING TIME

DIFFICULTY
○○○○○

OVEN TEMPERATURE

SOURCE

NUMBER OF SERVINGS

1 2 3 4 5 ....

°C

INGREDIENTS

_____
_____
_____
_____
_____
_____
_____

METHOD
_____
_____
_____
_____
_____
_____
_____
_____
_____
_____

NOTES
_____
_____
_____
_____
_____
_____

RECIPE ORIGIN
_____

RATING

☆☆☆☆☆

· ·

PREP TIME

:

COOKING TIME

DIFFICULTY

●●●●●

OVEN TEMPERATURE

_____

SOURCE

_____

NUMBER OF SERVINGS

1 2 3 4 5 ....

°C

INGREDIENTS

_____
_____
_____
_____
_____
_____
_____

___ ___

RECIPE ORIGIN

_____

NOTES

_____
_____
_____
_____
_____
_____
_____

METHOD

_____
_____
_____
_____
_____
_____
_____
_____
_____
_____
_____
_____

RATING
☆☆☆☆☆

· ·

PREP TIME

COOKING TIME

DIFFICULTY
○ ○ ○ ○ ○

OVEN TEMPERATURE

SOURCE
_____

NUMBER OF SERVINGS

1 2 3 4 5 ....

°C

INGREDIENTS

_____
_____
_____
_____
_____
_____
_____

METHOD

_____
_____
_____
_____
_____
_____
_____
_____
_____
_____
_____
_____
_____
_____

NOTES

_____
_____

_ _ _

RECIPE ORIGIN

_____

RATING

☆☆☆☆☆

· ·

PREP TIME

COOKING TIME

DIFFICULTY

OVEN TEMPERATURE

SOURCE

NUMBER OF SERVINGS

1 2 3 4 5 ....

℃

METHOD

INGREDIENTS

NOTES

RECIPE ORIGIN

RATING

☆☆☆☆☆

. . . .

:

PREP TIME

COOKING TIME

DIFFICULTY
○○○○○

OVEN TEMPERATURE

SOURCE

NUMBER OF SERVINGS

1 2 3 4 5 ....

°C

INGREDIENTS

METHOD

NOTES

RECIPE ORIGIN

RATING

☆☆☆☆☆

· ·

PREP TIME

COOKING TIME

DIFFICULTY

OVEN TEMPERATURE

SOURCE

NUMBER OF SERVINGS

1 2 3 4 5 ....

°C

INGREDIENTS

METHOD

NOTES

RECIPE ORIGIN

RATING

☆☆☆☆☆

· ·

PREP TIME

:

COOKING TIME

DIFFICULTY

● ● ● ● ●

OVEN TEMPERATURE

____

°C

SOURCE

____

NUMBER OF SERVINGS

1 2 3 4 5 ....

INGREDIENTS

_____

_____

_____

_____

_____

_____

_____

__ __

RECIPE ORIGIN

_____

NOTES

_____

_____

_____

_____

_____

_____

_____

METHOD

_____

_____

_____

_____

_____

_____

_____

_____

_____

_____

_____

_____

_____

_____

RATING

☆☆☆☆☆

....

PREP TIME

COOKING TIME

DIFFICULTY

○○○○○

OVEN TEMPERATURE

_____

SOURCE

_____

NUMBER OF SERVINGS

1 2 3 4 5 ....

°C

METHOD

_____
_____
_____
_____
_____
_____
_____
_____
_____
_____
_____

INGREDIENTS

_____
_____
_____
_____
_____
_____
_____

NOTES

_____
_____
_____
_____
_____
_____
_____
_____

_ _ _

RECIPE ORIGIN

_____

RATING

☆☆☆☆☆

- -

PREP TIME

COOKING TIME

DIFFICULTY

⚫⚫⚫⚫⚫

OVEN TEMPERATURE

°C

SOURCE

NUMBER OF SERVINGS

1 2 3 4 5 ....

INGREDIENTS

_____
_____
_____
_____
_____
_____
_____

METHOD

_____
_____
_____
_____
_____
_____
_____
_____
_____

NOTES

_____
_____
_____
_____
_____
_____

RECIPE ORIGIN

RATING
☆☆☆☆☆

· ·

PREP TIME

COOKING TIME

DIFFICULTY
○○○○○

OVEN TEMPERATURE

SOURCE

°C

NUMBER OF SERVINGS

1 2 3 4 5 ....

METHOD

INGREDIENTS

NOTES

RECIPE ORIGIN

RATING

☆☆☆☆☆

. . . .

PREP TIME

:

COOKING TIME

DIFFICULTY

OVEN TEMPERATURE

SOURCE

NUMBER OF SERVINGS

1 2 3 4 5 ....

°C

INGREDIENTS

METHOD

NOTES

RECIPE ORIGIN

RATING

☆☆☆☆☆

· ·

PREP TIME :

COOKING TIME

DIFFICULTY
○○○○○

OVEN TEMPERATURE

SOURCE

NUMBER OF SERVINGS

1 2 3 4 5 ....

°C

INGREDIENTS

_____

_____

_____

_____

_____

_____

_____

METHOD

_____

_____

_____

_____

_____

_____

_____

_____

_____

NOTES

_____

_____

_____

_____

_____

_____

_____

_____

_____

RECIPE ORIGIN

_____

RATING

☆☆☆☆☆

PREP TIME

COOKING TIME

DIFFICULTY

OVEN TEMPERATURE

SOURCE

_____

NUMBER OF SERVINGS

1 2 3 4 5 ....

°C

INGREDIENTS

_____

_____

_____

_____

_____

_____

_____

_____

METHOD

_____

_____

_____

_____

NOTES

_____

_____

__ __

_____

RECIPE ORIGIN

_____

_____

RATING
☆☆☆☆☆

....

PREP TIME

COOKING TIME

DIFFICULTY
○○○○○

OVEN TEMPERATURE
_____

SOURCE
_____

NUMBER OF SERVINGS

1 2 3 4 5 ....

°C

INGREDIENTS
_____
_____
_____
_____
_____
_____
_____

METHOD
_____
_____
_____
_____
_____
_____
_____
_____
_____
_____
_____

NOTES
_____
_____
_____

— — —

RECIPE ORIGIN
_____

RATING

☆☆☆☆☆

· ·

PREP TIME

COOKING TIME

DIFFICULTY

OVEN TEMPERATURE

SOURCE

NUMBER OF SERVINGS

1 2 3 4 5 ....

INGREDIENTS

METHOD

NOTES

RECIPE ORIGIN

°C

RATING
☆☆☆☆☆

....

PREP TIME

COOKING TIME

DIFFICULTY

OVEN TEMPERATURE

SOURCE

NUMBER OF SERVINGS

1 2 3 4 5 ....

°C

INGREDIENTS

METHOD

NOTES

RECIPE ORIGIN

RATING
☆☆☆☆☆

- -

:
PREP TIME

COOKING TIME

DIFFICULTY
○○○○○

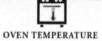

OVEN TEMPERATURE
———————

SOURCE
———————

NUMBER OF SERVINGS

1 2 3 4 5 ....

°c

INGREDIENTS
———————————
———————————
———————————
———————————
———————————
———————————
———————————

— —

RECIPE ORIGIN
———————————

METHOD
———————————————
———————————————
———————————————
———————————————
———————————————
———————————————
———————————————
———————————————
———————————————
———————————————
———————————————
———————————————

NOTES
———————
———————
———————
———————
———————
———————
———————
———————

RATING
☆☆☆☆☆

....

PREP TIME

COOKING TIME

DIFFICULTY
○○○○○

OVEN TEMPERATURE

SOURCE
_____

NUMBER OF SERVINGS

1 2 3 4 5 ....

°C

INGREDIENTS
_____
_____
_____
_____
_____
_____
_____

METHOD
_____
_____
_____
_____
_____
_____
_____
_____

NOTES
_____
_____
_____
_____
_____
_____
_____

— —

RECIPE ORIGIN
_____

RATING

☆☆☆☆☆

....

PREP TIME

COOKING TIME

DIFFICULTY
●●●●●

OVEN TEMPERATURE

SOURCE

NUMBER OF SERVINGS

1 2 3 4 5 ....

°c

INGREDIENTS

METHOD

NOTES

RECIPE ORIGIN

RATING

☆☆☆☆☆

....

PREP TIME

COOKING TIME

DIFFICULTY

⬤⬤⬤⬤⬤

OVEN TEMPERATURE

°C

SOURCE

NUMBER OF SERVINGS

1 2 3 4 5 ....

INGREDIENTS

_____
_____
_____
_____
_____
_____
_____

METHOD

_____
_____
_____
_____
_____
_____
_____
_____
_____
_____
_____
_____
_____
_____
_____

NOTES

_____
_____
_____
_____
_____
_____

RECIPE ORIGIN

_____

RATING

☆☆☆☆☆

· ·

PREP TIME

COOKING TIME

DIFFICULTY

OVEN TEMPERATURE

SOURCE

NUMBER OF SERVINGS

1 2 3 4 5 ....

°C

INGREDIENTS

_____

_____

_____

_____

_____

_____

_____

METHOD

_____

_____

_____

_____

_____

_____

_____

_____

_____

NOTES

_____

_____

_____

_____

_____

_____

_____

RECIPE ORIGIN

_____

_____

_____

_____

RATING
☆☆☆☆☆

· ·

PREP TIME

COOKING TIME

DIFFICULTY
◯◯◯◯

OVEN TEMPERATURE

SOURCE
_____

NUMBER OF SERVINGS

1 2 3 4 5 ....

℃

INGREDIENTS

_____
_____
_____
_____
_____
_____
_____

METHOD

_____
_____
_____
_____
_____
_____
_____
_____
_____
_____
_____

NOTES

_____
_____
_____
_____
_____
_____

___ ___

RECIPE ORIGIN

_____

RATING

☆☆☆☆☆

· ·

:

PREP TIME

COOKING TIME

DIFFICULTY
●●●●

OVEN TEMPERATURE

SOURCE

NUMBER OF SERVINGS

1 2 3 4 5 ....

°C

INGREDIENTS

METHOD

NOTES

RECIPE ORIGIN

RATING

☆☆☆☆☆

· ·

PREP TIME

COOKING TIME

DIFFICULTY

OVEN TEMPERATURE

SOURCE
_____

°C

NUMBER OF SERVINGS

1 2 3 4 5 ....

INGREDIENTS

_____
_____
_____
_____
_____
_____
_____

_ _ _

RECIPE ORIGIN
_____

METHOD

_____
_____
_____
_____
_____
_____
_____
_____
_____
_____
_____
_____
_____
_____
_____

NOTES

_____
_____
_____
_____
_____
_____
_____
_____

RATING
☆☆☆☆☆

PREP TIME

COOKING TIME

DIFFICULTY
○○○○○

OVEN TEMPERATURE
____

SOURCE
____

NUMBER OF SERVINGS

1 2 3 4 5 ....

°C

INGREDIENTS
____
____
____
____
____
____
____

METHOD
____
____
____
____
____
____
____
____
____
____
____
____
____
____

NOTES
____
____
____

RECIPE ORIGIN
_____

RATING

☆☆☆☆☆

....

PREP TIME

COOKING TIME

DIFFICULTY
○○○○○

OVEN TEMPERATURE

°C

SOURCE

NUMBER OF SERVINGS

1 2 3 4 5 ....

INGREDIENTS

METHOD

NOTES

RECIPE ORIGIN

RATING

☆☆☆☆☆

....

PREP TIME

COOKING TIME

DIFFICULTY
○○○○○

OVEN TEMPERATURE

SOURCE
_____

NUMBER OF SERVINGS

1 2 3 4 5 ....

°C

INGREDIENTS

_____
_____
_____
_____
_____
_____
_____

RECIPE ORIGIN
_____

NOTES

_____
_____
_____
_____
_____
_____
_____

METHOD

_____
_____
_____
_____
_____
_____
_____
_____
_____
_____
_____
_____
_____
_____

RATING

☆☆☆☆☆

· ·

PREP TIME

COOKING TIME

DIFFICULTY

OVEN TEMPERATURE

SOURCE

NUMBER OF SERVINGS

1 2 3 4 5 ....

°C

METHOD

INGREDIENTS

_____

_____

_____

_____

_____

_____

_____

_____

NOTES

_____

_____

_____

_____

_____

_____

_____

_____

RECIPE ORIGIN

RATING
☆☆☆☆☆

- -

PREP TIME

COOKING TIME

DIFFICULTY
○○○○

OVEN TEMPERATURE
_____

SOURCE
_____

NUMBER OF SERVINGS

1 2 3 4 5 ....

°C

INGREDIENTS
_____
_____
_____
_____
_____
_____
_____

METHOD
_____
_____
_____
_____
_____
_____
_____
_____

NOTES
_____
_____
_____
_____
_____
_____
_____
_____

— —

RECIPE ORIGIN
_____

RATING
☆☆☆☆☆

. . . .

PREP TIME

COOKING TIME

DIFFICULTY

OVEN TEMPERATURE

SOURCE

°C

NUMBER OF SERVINGS

1 2 3 4 5 ....

INGREDIENTS

METHOD

NOTES

RECIPE ORIGIN

RATING
☆☆☆☆☆

....

PREP TIME

COOKING TIME

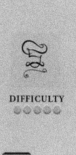

DIFFICULTY
○○○○○

OVEN TEMPERATURE
_____

SOURCE
_____

NUMBER OF SERVINGS

1 2 3 4 5 ....

℃

INGREDIENTS

_____
_____
_____
_____
_____
_____
_____
_____

__ __ __

RECIPE ORIGIN

_____

METHOD

_____
_____
_____
_____
_____
_____
_____
_____
_____
_____
_____
_____
_____
_____

NOTES

_____
_____
_____
_____
_____
_____
_____
_____

RATING

☆☆☆☆☆

....

PREP TIME

COOKING TIME

DIFFICULTY

OVEN TEMPERATURE

SOURCE

NUMBER OF SERVINGS

1 2 3 4 5 ....

°C

INGREDIENTS

METHOD

NOTES

RECIPE ORIGIN

RATING
☆☆☆☆☆

....

:
PREP TIME

COOKING TIME

DIFFICULTY
○ ○ ○ ○ ○

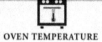
OVEN TEMPERATURE
————

SOURCE
————

NUMBER OF SERVINGS

1 2 3 4 5 ....

°C

INGREDIENTS

————————————————
————————————————
————————————————
————————————————
————————————————
————————————————
————————————————

— — —

RECIPE ORIGIN

————————

NOTES

————————
————————
————————
————————
————————
————————
————————
————————

METHOD

————————————————
————————————————
————————————————
————————————————
————————————————
————————————————
————————————————
————————————————
————————————————
————————————————
————————————————
————————————————
————————————————
————————————————
————————————————
————————————————

RATING
☆☆☆☆☆

....

PREP TIME

COOKING TIME

DIFFICULTY

OVEN TEMPERATURE
_____

SOURCE
_____

NUMBER OF SERVINGS

1 2 3 4 5 ....

℃

INGREDIENTS

_____
_____
_____
_____
_____
_____
_____

METHOD

_____
_____
_____
_____
_____
_____
_____
_____
_____
_____
_____
_____

NOTES

_____
_____
_____
_____
_____
_____
_____

— —

RECIPE ORIGIN

_____

RATING

☆☆☆☆☆

· ·

PREP TIME

COOKING TIME

DIFFICULTY

○○○○○

OVEN TEMPERATURE

SOURCE

NUMBER OF SERVINGS

1 2 3 4 5 ....

°C

INGREDIENTS

METHOD

NOTES

RECIPE ORIGIN

RATING

☆☆☆☆☆

....

PREP TIME

COOKING TIME

DIFFICULTY

OVEN TEMPERATURE

SOURCE

NUMBER OF SERVINGS

1 2 3 4 5 ....

°C

INGREDIENTS

METHOD

NOTES

RECIPE ORIGIN

RATING
☆☆☆☆☆

....

PREP TIME

COOKING TIME

DIFFICULTY
○○○○

OVEN TEMPERATURE

SOURCE

NUMBER OF SERVINGS

1 2 3 4 5 ....

°C

INGREDIENTS

METHOD

NOTES

RECIPE ORIGIN

RATING

☆☆☆☆☆

· ·

:

PREP TIME

COOKING TIME

DIFFICULTY

○○○○

OVEN TEMPERATURE

SOURCE

NUMBER OF SERVINGS

1 2 3 4 5 ....

°C

INGREDIENTS

_____

_____

_____

_____

_____

_____

_____

METHOD

NOTES

RECIPE ORIGIN

RATING
☆☆☆☆☆

....

:

PREP TIME

COOKING TIME

DIFFICULTY
● ○ ○ ○ ○

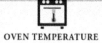

OVEN TEMPERATURE
_____

SOURCE
_____

NUMBER OF SERVINGS

1 2 3 4 5 ....

°C

INGREDIENTS

_____
_____
_____
_____
_____
_____
_____

— __

RECIPE ORIGIN

_____

METHOD

_____
_____
_____
_____
_____
_____
_____
_____
_____
_____
_____
_____
_____

NOTES

_____
_____
_____
_____
_____
_____
_____

RATING
☆☆☆☆☆

....

⏰
PREP TIME

🕐
COOKING TIME

DIFFICULTY
○○○○○

🍳
OVEN TEMPERATURE
_____

SOURCE
_____

NUMBER OF SERVINGS

1 2 3 4 5 ....

INGREDIENTS
_____
_____
_____
_____
_____
_____
_____
_____

__ __

RECIPE ORIGIN
_____

°C

METHOD
_____
_____
_____
_____
_____
_____
_____
_____
_____
_____
_____
_____
_____
_____
_____
_____

📝
NOTES
_____
_____
_____
_____
_____
_____
_____
_____

RATING

☆☆☆☆☆

. . . .

PREP TIME

COOKING TIME

DIFFICULTY

OVEN TEMPERATURE

SOURCE

NUMBER OF SERVINGS

1 2 3 4 5 ....

°C

INGREDIENTS

METHOD

NOTES

RECIPE ORIGIN

RATING

☆☆☆☆☆

....

PREP TIME

COOKING TIME

DIFFICULTY
○○○○○

OVEN TEMPERATURE

SOURCE

NUMBER OF SERVINGS

1 2 3 4 5 ....

°C

INGREDIENTS

METHOD

NOTES

RECIPE ORIGIN

RATING
☆☆☆☆☆

··

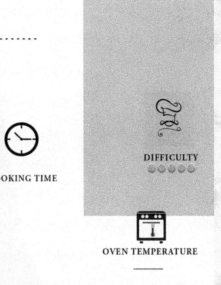

PREP TIME

COOKING TIME

DIFFICULTY
⦾⦾⦾⦾⦾

OVEN TEMPERATURE
_____

°C

SOURCE
_____

NUMBER OF SERVINGS

1 2 3 4 5 ....

INGREDIENTS

_____
_____
_____
_____
_____
_____
_____

— — —

RECIPE ORIGIN
_____

NOTES

_____
_____
_____
_____
_____
_____
_____
_____

METHOD

_____
_____
_____
_____
_____
_____
_____
_____
_____
_____
_____
_____
_____
_____

RATING

☆☆☆☆☆

....

PREP TIME

COOKING TIME

DIFFICULTY

OVEN TEMPERATURE

SOURCE

NUMBER OF SERVINGS

1 2 3 4 5 ....

℃

INGREDIENTS

METHOD

NOTES

RECIPE ORIGIN

RATING

☆☆☆☆☆

PREP TIME

COOKING TIME

DIFFICULTY
○○○○○

OVEN TEMPERATURE
_____

°C

SOURCE
_____

NUMBER OF SERVINGS

1 2 3 4 5 ....

INGREDIENTS
_____
_____
_____
_____
_____
_____
_____

__ __

RECIPE ORIGIN
_____

METHOD
_____
_____
_____
_____
_____
_____
_____
_____
_____
_____
_____
_____

NOTES
_____
_____
_____
_____
_____
_____

RATING
☆☆☆☆☆

. . . .

PREP TIME

COOKING TIME

DIFFICULTY
●●●●●

OVEN TEMPERATURE
_____

SOURCE
_____

NUMBER OF SERVINGS

1 2 3 4 5 ....

INGREDIENTS
_____
_____
_____
_____
_____
_____
_____
_____

__ _ __

RECIPE ORIGIN
_____

NOTES
_____
_____
_____
_____
_____
_____

METHOD
_____
_____
_____
_____
_____
_____
_____
_____
_____
_____
_____
_____
_____
_____

℃

RATING

☆☆☆☆☆

....

PREP TIME

COOKING TIME

DIFFICULTY
●●●●●

OVEN TEMPERATURE
_____

SOURCE
_____

NUMBER OF SERVINGS

1 2 3 4 5 ....

°C

INGREDIENTS

_____
_____
_____
_____
_____
_____
_____

NOTES

_____

RECIPE ORIGIN

_____

METHOD

_____
_____
_____
_____
_____
_____
_____
_____
_____
_____
_____
_____
_____
_____

RATING

☆☆☆☆☆

....

PREP TIME

COOKING TIME

DIFFICULTY
○○○○○

OVEN TEMPERATURE

SOURCE

NUMBER OF SERVINGS

1 2 3 4 5 ....

°C

INGREDIENTS

_____

_____

_____

_____

_____

_____

_____

METHOD

_____

_____

_____

_____

_____

_____

_____

_____

_____

_____

NOTES

_____

_____

_____

_____

RECIPE ORIGIN

_____

_____

_____

_____

_____

_____

_____

_____

RATING

☆☆☆☆☆

....

PREP TIME

COOKING TIME

DIFFICULTY

OVEN TEMPERATURE
—————

SOURCE
—————

NUMBER OF SERVINGS

1 2 3 4 5 ....

METHOD
_____
_____
_____
_____

INGREDIENTS
_____
_____
_____
_____
_____
_____
_____

NOTES
_____
_____

°C

_____
_____
_____
_____
_____
_____

—— ——

RECIPE ORIGIN
—————————

RATING

☆☆☆☆☆

....

PREP TIME

COOKING TIME

DIFFICULTY
○ ○ ○ ○ ○

OVEN TEMPERATURE

SOURCE

NUMBER OF SERVINGS

1 2 3 4 5 ....

°C

INGREDIENTS

_____

_____

_____

_____

_____

_____

_____

— —

RECIPE ORIGIN

_____

METHOD

_____

_____

_____

_____

_____

_____

_____

_____

_____

_____

_____

_____

_____

_____

_____

NOTES

_____

_____

_____

_____

_____

_____

RATING

☆☆☆☆☆

....

PREP TIME

COOKING TIME

DIFFICULTY
⬤⬤⬤⬤⬤

OVEN TEMPERATURE
_____

SOURCE
_____

NUMBER OF SERVINGS

1 2 3 4 5 ....

°C

INGREDIENTS

_____
_____
_____
_____
_____
_____
_____

METHOD

_____
_____
_____
_____
_____
_____
_____
_____
_____
_____
_____
_____
_____

NOTES

_____
_____
_____
_____
_____
_____

— —

RECIPE ORIGIN

_____

RATING

☆☆☆☆☆

· ·

PREP TIME

COOKING TIME

DIFFICULTY

OVEN TEMPERATURE

SOURCE

NUMBER OF SERVINGS

1 2 3 4 5 ....

°C

INGREDIENTS

_____

_____

_____

_____

_____

_____

_____

NOTES

_____

_____

_____

_____

METHOD

_____

_____

_____

_____

_____

_____

_____

_____

_____

_____

_____

_____

_____

_____

RECIPE ORIGIN

_____

RATING

☆☆☆☆☆

....

PREP TIME

COOKING TIME

DIFFICULTY

SOURCE

OVEN TEMPERATURE

NUMBER OF SERVINGS

1 2 3 4 5 ....

INGREDIENTS

METHOD

NOTES

RECIPE ORIGIN

RATING

☆☆☆☆☆

....

PREP TIME

COOKING TIME

DIFFICULTY

OVEN TEMPERATURE

SOURCE

NUMBER OF SERVINGS

1 2 3 4 5 ....

°C

INGREDIENTS

METHOD

NOTES

RECIPE ORIGIN

CPSIA information can be obtained
at www.ICGtesting.com
Printed in the USA
LVHW021926060121
675853LV00022B/1270